Dedications

To my children Luke and Lauryn

for your growing inspiration

Kids Backs 4 The Future (KB4TF), created for
a healthier lifestyle

© Written by Lyndee Oscar

ISBN-13:978-1517464363

Illustrated by Shermain Philip

*"As a registered osteopath for over 23
years, it is my responsibility to use my
knowledge of back care to protect the younger
generation from unnecessary musculoskeletal
risk.
Prevention is always better than cure"*

Lyndee Oscar MSc., BSc (Hons).,D.O

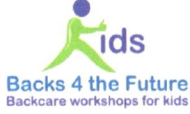

Backs 4 the Future
Backcare workshops for kids

www.kidsback4thefuture.co.uk

Founder of KB4TF

Helping Kids Become Back Wise

"Back pain is now the world's leading cause of human disability and together with related musculoskeletal conditions, accounts for a quarter of UK sickness absence. Orienting children towards positive health-related beliefs and behaviours is undoubtedly the most legitimate activity of our public health responsibility. Whatever good we can do for health is best achieved in childhood.
 This book gives children a good emphasis on physical activity as well as a physical awareness approach"

Dr Adam Al-Kashi, Head of Research and Education for BackCare – the UK's national back and neck pain charity

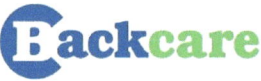

Our Penstripe back health page in school planners/reading books are supporting Backcare and Kids Backs 4 The Future in helping raise awareness of back care at schoolage

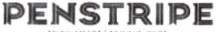

"In our modern world, little attention is paid to the damage caused to developing bones by modern lifestyles. Teaching schoolchildren to be aware of the impact ordinary activities in their daily lives can have on their bodies is vitally important to ensuring our children grow up with healthy backs. This book is a fantastic addition to any school library to inform children at an early age, before the developing bones in the spine and muscles are damaged from activities such as poor postures, reduced activity and carrying loads incorrectly"

Janet Fay Director

Marathons School Bag Specialist

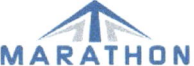

Sportsafe UK are pleased to support Kids Backs 4 The Future in keeping kids active.

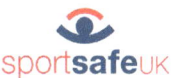

This is a play and learn book about the muscles *(say: Mus-els)* we use.

Muscles are all around our body. Our muscles help us to move around and are attached to our bones by tendons *(say:Ten-dons)* and ligaments *(say: Lig a-ments)* attach our bones together.

Thanks to our muscles, we can jump, run, play games, smile, eat and breathe.

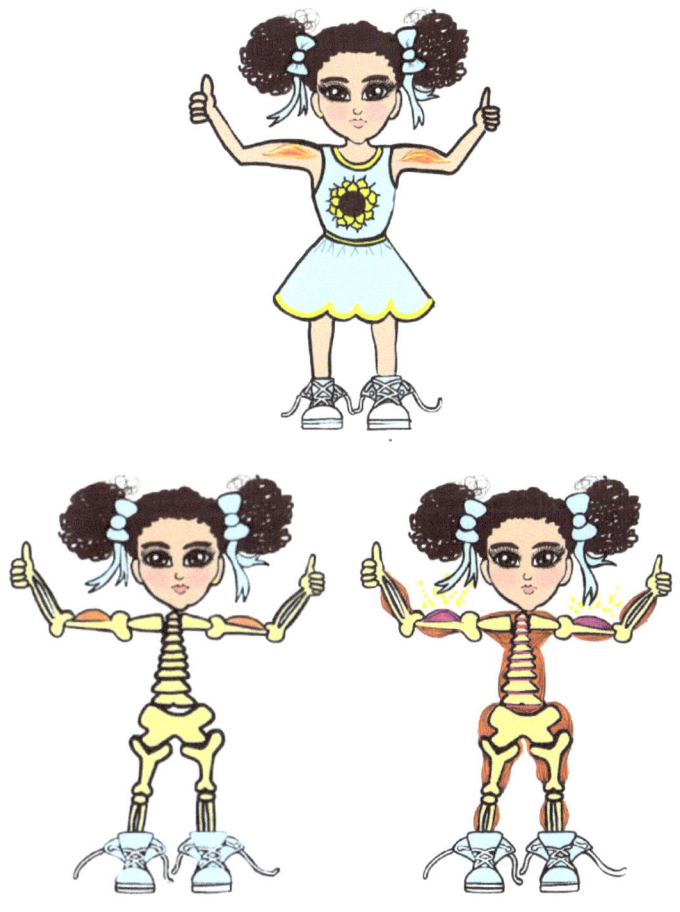

Our Muscles

There are over 600 muscles in the body.

40 percent of our body is muscle.

(That's nearly half of our body!)

The smallest muscle is in the ear and the largest one is in the bottom.

The brain tells the muscles how and when to move.

Keeping our muscles moving, by stretching and being active is very important.

Watch me and watch the muscles I use!

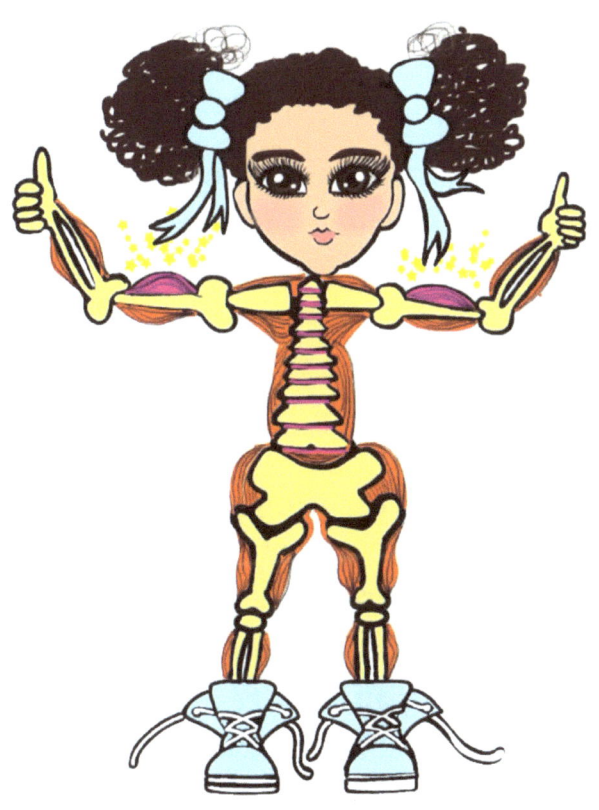

Different muscles

Your tongue is a muscle too.
Stick your tongue out and
wiggle it around.

Watch how the muscles on
your face move.

Your heart muscle is called
Cardiac
(Say: Kar de-ak).
Every time you breath you
use your heart muscle.

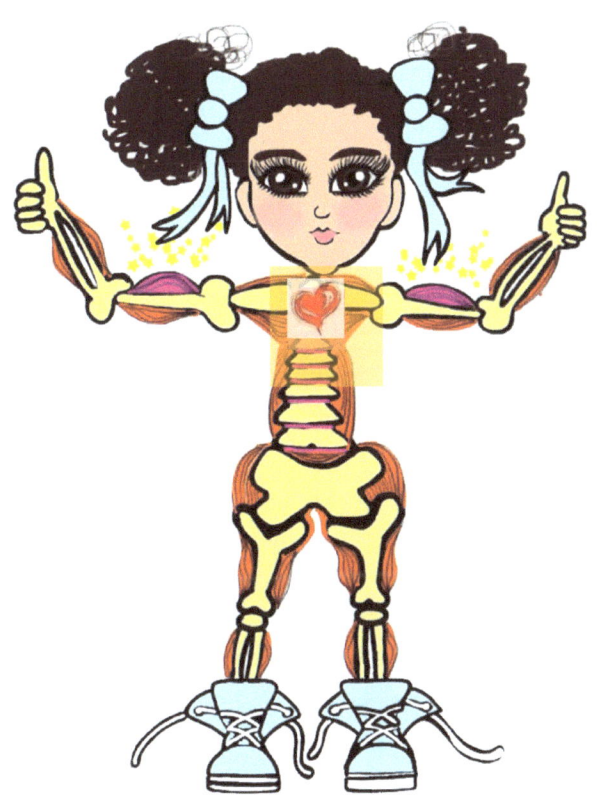

When you Cat Stretch, you use mainly the muscles in your shoulders, arms and chest.

When I wake up I do a big, big Cat Stretch.

I call it a Cat Stretch because it looks like a Cat stretching!

Watch me and watch the muscles I use!

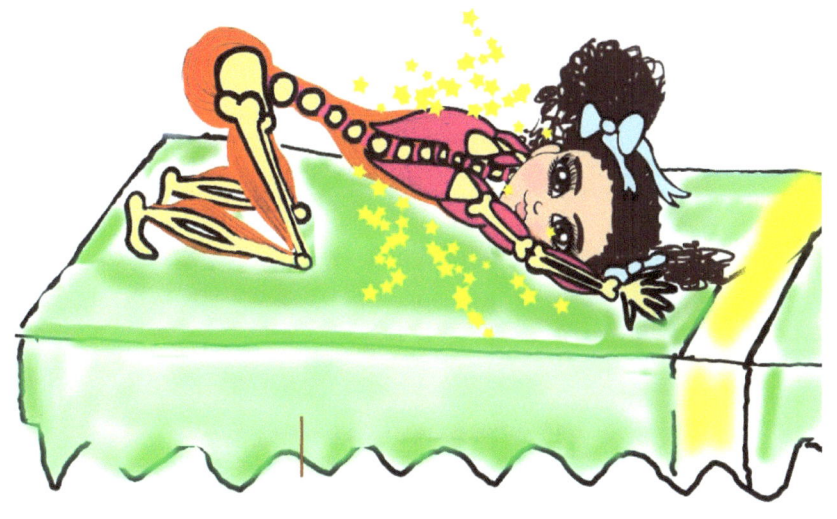

When you yawn, you use mainly the muscles in your arms and your face.

After I cat stretch, I do a big, big yawn.

Watch me and watch the muscles I use!

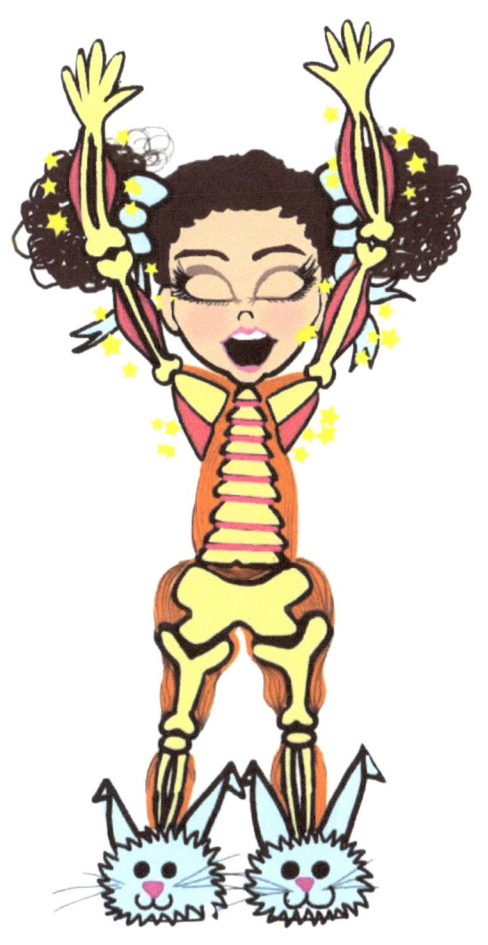

When you brush your teeth, you use mainly the muscles in your hands, arms and shoulders.

In the morning I go into the bathroom and brush my teeth.

Watch me and watch the muscles I use!

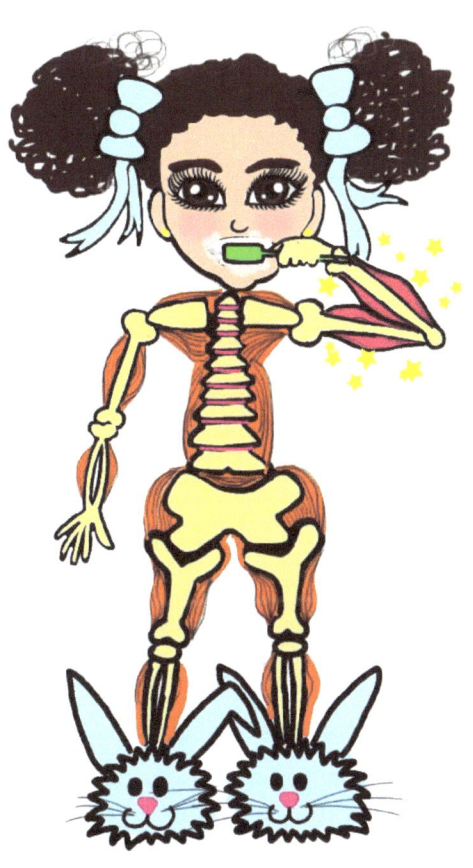

When you wash your face, you use mainly the muscles in your head, neck and shoulders.

After I brush my teeth, I wash my face.

Watch me and watch the muscles I use!

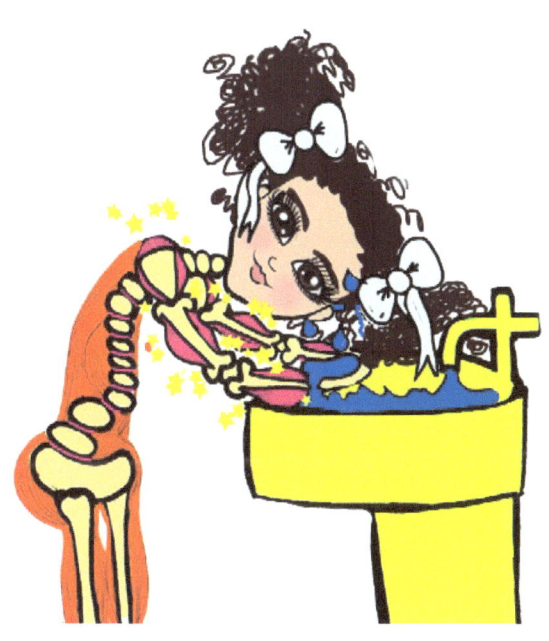

When you reach for your clothes, you use mainly the muscles in your hands, arms, shoulders and legs.

I reach for my clothes.

Watch me and watch the muscles I use!

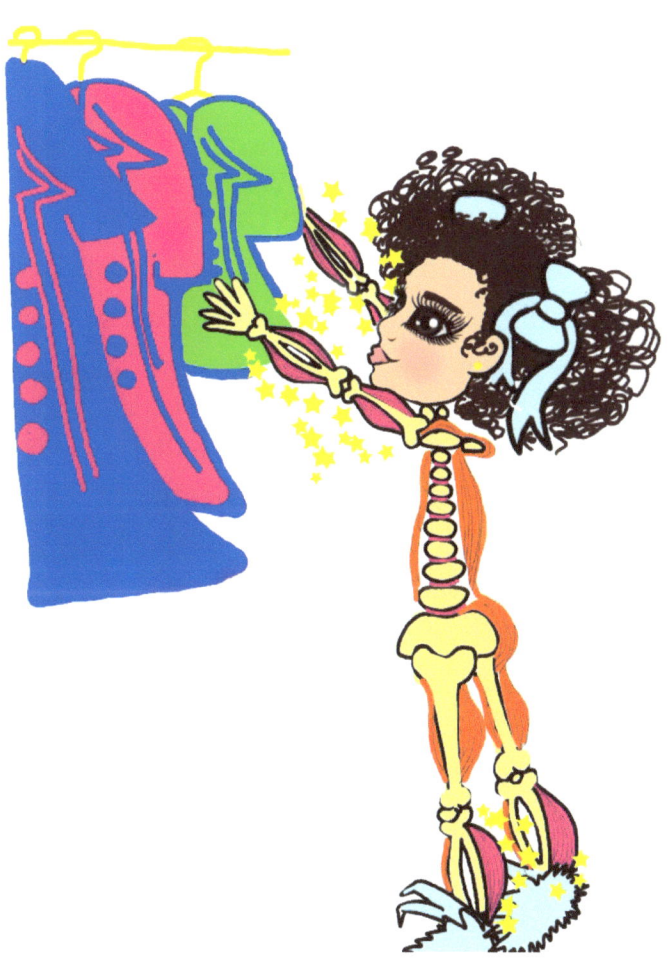

When you go down the stairs, you use mainly the muscles in your hands, arms, shoulders and legs.

Then I go down the stairs holding on to the banister.

Watch me and watch the muscles I use!

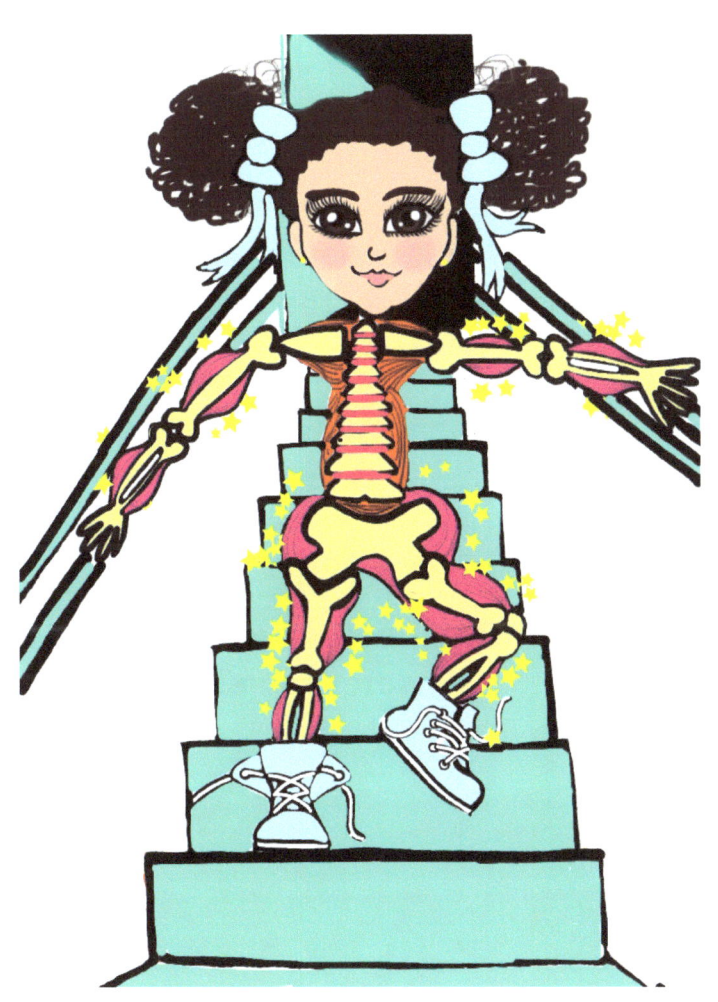

When you sit down at the table, you use mainly the muscles in your legs and toes.

I sit down to eat my breakfast. I play touching toes with my brother under the table.

Watch me and watch the muscles I use!

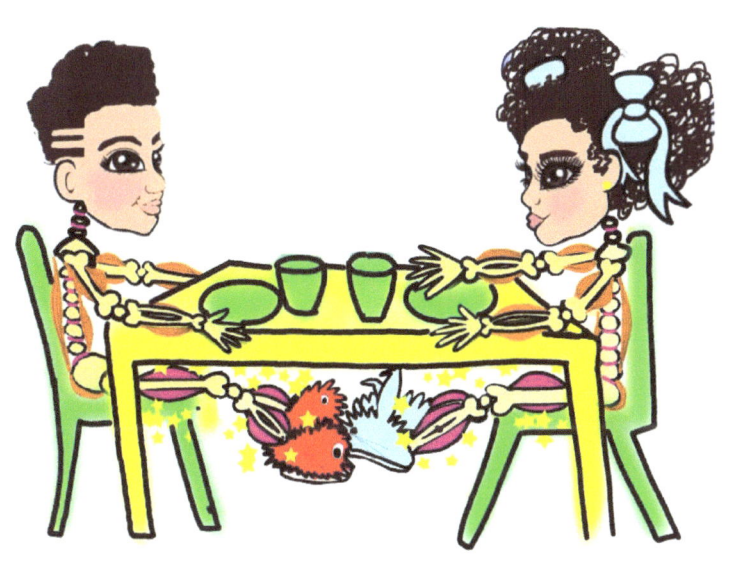

When you reach for your coat and bag, you use mainly the muscles in your arms, shoulders, legs and feet.

I reach for my coat and bag before I go to school.

Watch me and watch the muscles I use!

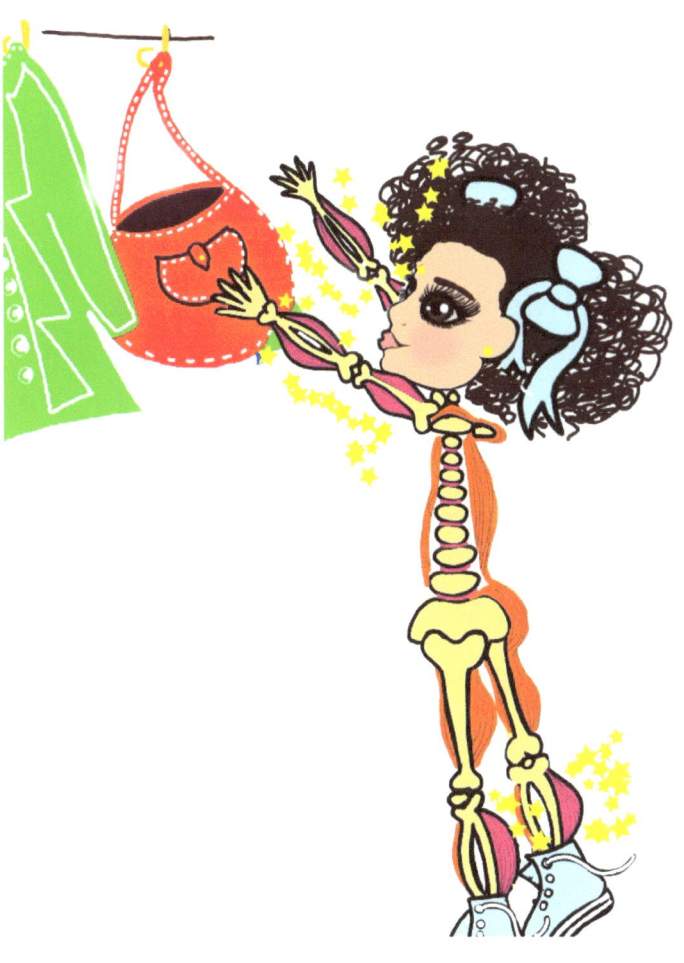

When you walk, you use mainly all of your muscles.

I briskly walk to school with my mummy.

Watch me and watch the muscles I use!

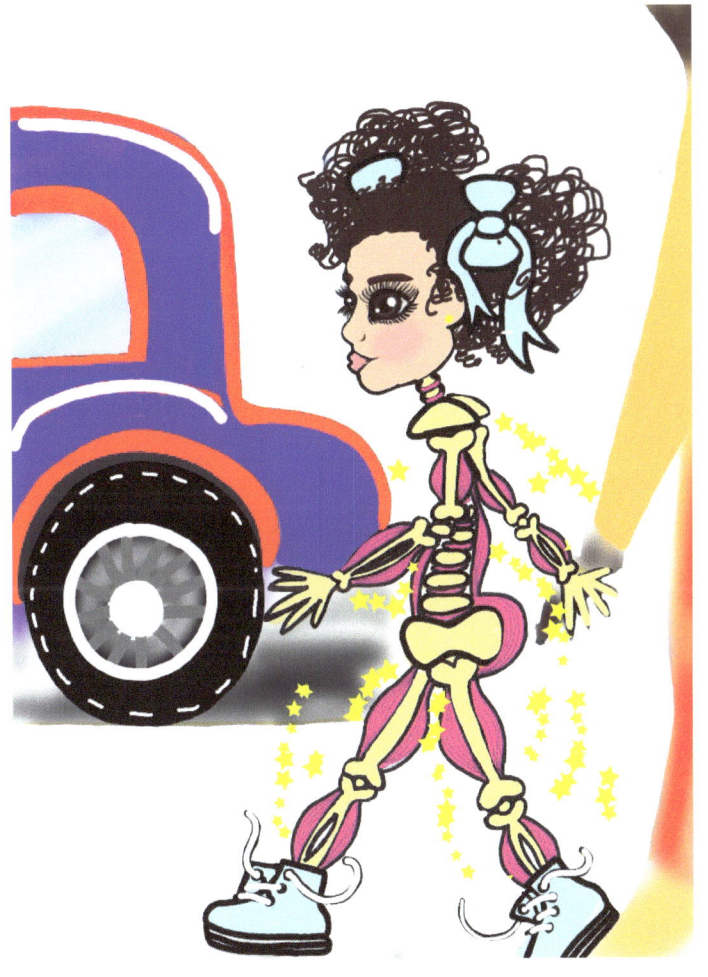

To keep your muscles in good shape you need to:

Eat healthy to grow well.

Keep your muscles moving by keeping active and stretching.

Use your face muscles often to smile and be happy.

Make sure you get plenty of rest and sleep.

Exercises makes you feel good, relaxes your muscles and helps get rid of stress.

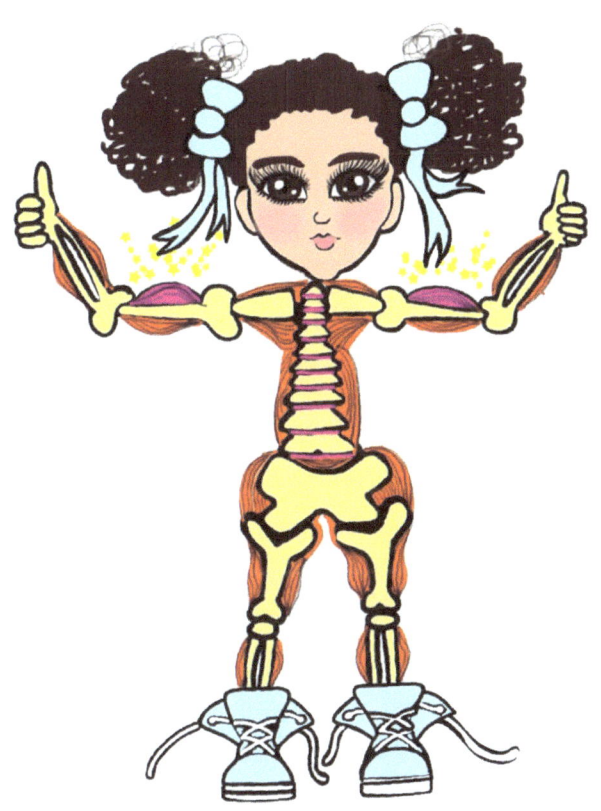

10 fun play and learn things to do after reading this book

Find the answers in the book

1. Our muscles-What do your muscles help you to do? Show us!
2. How many muscles in your body? What percentage of your body is muscle?
3. Is your heart a muscle? -what is another name for your heart muscle?
4. Where is the smallest muscle in your body? Point to it!
5. Ligaments – What do ligaments attach together? Point to any ligament!
6. Tendons – What do tendons attach together? Point to any tendon!
7. What part of the body tells the muscles how and when to move? Point to it on your body.
8. Stretch out and smile. Do a few of the stretches in the book-Watch and feel the muscles you use! Stretching feels good!
9. What does exercises do? What exercises do you do? Tell everyone!
10. What can you do to keep your muscles in good shape? Show us!

Well done and make sure you do these things!

For more support to help you stay Back Wise

download our Back Wise posters and visit www.kidsbacks4thefuture.co.uk

Also in the series

Look out for

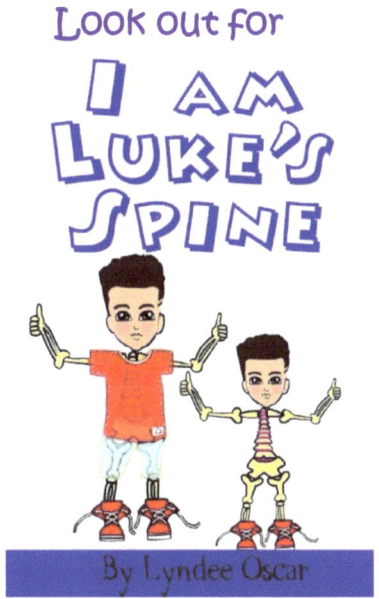

I AM LUKE'S SPINE

By Lyndee Oscar

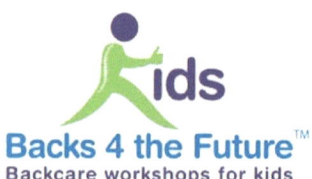

Backs 4 the Future™
Backcare workshops for kids

Kids achieve an A+ in being Back Wise

www.kidsbacks4thefuture.co.uk

SIT WELL

An S shape posture is a good healthy posture. It will improve what you do and reduce any pain or discomfort.

STRETCH WELL

Remember to take short regular breaks. Stand up, stretch out your back and hand muscles to avoid discomfort and stiffness. Adjust your position often.

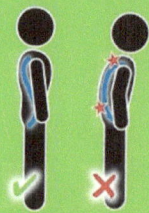

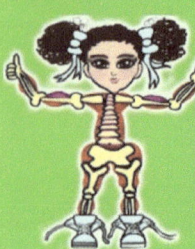

and remember to..

FEEL WELL!!

Keeping active, exercising and eating healthy will help you to grow well!

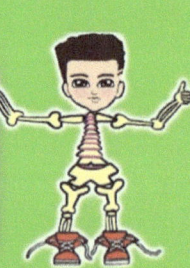

READ WELL

Keep your head upright and avoid looking down at your book, tablet or smart device as this will cause pain in your neck, shoulders and back.

CARRY WELL

Keep your body balanced, stand or sit upright and carry your bag on both shoulders.

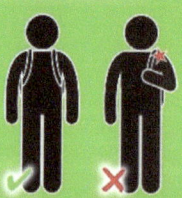

- Practice these Back Wise tips today to prevent back pain tomorrow
- Keep Active

- Eat and drink well to grow well
- Keep happy
- Let someone know if you have back pain

In support of 2015 **Backcare** National Awareness Class Campaign focussing on back pain in young people